DIABETIC HEATH REGENERATION PLAN

Joseph Lee

Dragon KI Corporation

Email: kaiszen76@gmail.com

Vreeland President and CEO of Black Dragon KI Corporation

This document is a basis on understanding what Diabetes actually is, what causes it to happen and the differences between type 1 and type 2, as well included is a detoxification process in which the problems that cause diabetes can be removed from the body to help to possibly bring a cure for Diabetes, the idea is once the problem that caused the disease is eliminated then the disease itself can be completely eradicated from the body.

Diabetic heath regeneration plan for Diabetes type 1 and 2

This document will first outline the differences between diabetes type 1 and 2 and then provide a diet and exercise routine for healing, with what each type should avoid and what they should be eating. Since this is a professional work up on the diseases there will be references included along with my own conclusion toward the removal of this destructive disease. References will be from Scholarly resources found on google or the Library of the University of Phoenix. To begin this document we first need to make it clear that no disease is incurable except within the mind, so with part of this program we will be instating parts of what is known to be the "Biology of Belief" brought back to life by Dr. Bruce Lipton.

What is type 1 diabetes and how is it caused:

Type 1 diabetes in simple terms is when a person cannot consume sugar, if the glucose level raises to high then the person can go into shock and be at risk of death, so definitively the person my forgo eating sugar and consume vegetables that help to lower the sugar levels. This can be related to the non-diabetic form of the disease known as hyperglycemia. From the article written at https://www.nhs.uk/conditions/type-1-diabetes/ type 1 diabetes is an immune system disorder that quote "can't be cure" basically the disease is where the immune system attacks the pancreatic cells that deliver insulin to the body's cells so that they can absorb the incoming glucose and help to build the cellular energy for development of the body structure, such as gaining weight. For now it is suggested that one maintains the sugar levels as much as possible. Some research suggests that lowered levels of Vitamin D intake can help be a leading cause toward this disease.

Possible causes of type 1 diabetes according to research papers:

- Lack of Vitamin D
- Psychological (prenatal or postnatal stress)

- Environmental impact (such as over chemical exposure)
- The Overload and accelerator hypothesis
- Autoimmune Disorders
- Antigenic responses (allergic reactions)
- Possible Viral infections

What is type 2 diabetes and how is it caused:

In the definition and understanding of type 2 diabetes we must look toward hypoglycemia and the fact that the pancreas cannot keep up with the production of insulin in order to help keep the blood glucose levels normal. This causes the sugars aka glucose to remain within the blood and to not be used for energy. The causes of this problem can be brought on from:

Possible causes of type 2 Diabetes, according to research papers:

- Psychological Factors
- Environmental impact
- Poor diet
- Lack of exercise
- Excessive smoking

- Antigenic Reactions (allergic reactions

What is Diabetes mellitus and how is it caused:

This is the general terminology for both types of diabetes the differences are shifted to type 1 and type 2 based on how the levels of sugars are processed or not processed within the body with the insulin created within the pancreas. Type 1 is related to hyperglycemia or the fact that pancreas has completely stopped creating cells to produce insulin in the body to help regulate the levels of glucose. Type 2 is where the pancreas still produces the cells but not enough to keep up with the levels of sugars in the body. There are occasions when a very dangerous combination of both type 1 and type 2 which must be regulated through medication as of today's date there are no known cures for Type 1 diabetes based on the medical worlds determination, now whether this is due to wanting to keep patients. Basically stated no cure for type 1 diabetes, has ever been found to date due to the fact of trying to cure diabetes itself rather than looking at the known causes of it and treating them.

Understanding what Insulin is:

Insulin is a hormone created by the pancreas in the body that helps to transmute sugar into usable glucose that the cells of the body can take and use for production of energy for such things as building muscles, helping to strengthen bones, and production of the substance used for protecting the joints in the body known as cartilage which contains Synovial membrane and Synovial fluid as well as small sacs of fluid known as Bursae that are located between the muscles, tendons, ligaments and bones to help smoother movement though the cartilage Synovial membrane and Synovial fluid are the main part of the joints and once they start to wear down from the inability to repair them naturally this creates joint problems such as arthritis. Without the insulin there is no way that the body can use the glucose in the blood stream to help maintain the organs or joints in the body. So the lie of stripping sugar from your body is good is completely a lie in most cases, though in the case of type 1 diabetes it is necessary to remove the sugars till the pancreas can be repaired and a normal production of inulin can be produced naturally within the body.

Type 2 diabetes is the easiest to deal with, when it comes to cures just avoiding certain things such as genetically modified foods, conventionally produced foods (meaning those that use chemical pesticides and herbicides), Food Chemicals such as colorants and preservatives and artificial sweeteners, proper exercise in the diet. This alone can help improve or even get rid of type 2 diabetes, whereas with other factors included such as psychological factors with depression must also be treated without condemnation of the factors causing the problem, the people must be aware of the unconscious developed thoughts and remove them replacing them with better minded thoughts, the Chakra system relation to this is the solar plexus chakra.

With Environmental factors we have to deal with are the current allopathic medical staff and the use of destructive chemicals within the current state of medicine. Also the pollution of chemicals,

EMF's as well as can be a cause of most disease problems due to the genetic manipulation that can be caused through the consumption of the genetically modified foods as well as vaccinations to cause corruption of the DNA which leads toward RNA delivering corrupted sequences to the cells of the body which can cause cell death as well as mutation. Such can occur with Diabetes type one, a form of genetic mutation within the immune system directly causing the white blood cells to receive information to attack the pancreas and the cells released by the pancreas destroying them and shutting down the pancreas preventing the production of any more insulin in the body, thus throwing the body into a state of shock. As stated above the problems that can cause this are viral, psychological, excessive weight gain and excessive weight loss, environmental factors, and antigenic responses also known as allergic reactions. So now that the basis of the cause of the disease and what happens during the disease is covered we can move toward helping to possibly cure the disease as well has helping to prevent the disease within the future.

Type 1 diabetes disease causes, and cures to help remove the problem and prevent it in the future.

For autoimmune disorders: an autoimmune disorder happens when a corrupted DNA strand sends out RNA to cells giving the wrong signals to organs, other cells and the lymphatic system, among other places to attack or not accept the original coding within the body and reject such things like sugar. Autoimmune diseases are also related to antigenic responses, such as allergies and are governed by the immune system are sent signals not only from the DNA but the nervous system or rather neurological system within the body to cause damage and prevent the organs and bodies systems from working.

Viral problems causing diabetes type one problems again relate back to the autoimmune disorders from the virus taking over and corrupting the signals from the DNA and nervous system to cause problems and the development of diabetes type 1. In curing a problem that has been caused by a virus one must cure the virus then remove the problems caused by the virus.

Psychological problems that cause diabetes type 1, one must remove the psychological problems first then correct the diet, in removing the psychological problems we can look toward the chakras such as the solar plexus chakra which is connected truly to the pancreas.

A lack of vitamin D there are 2 case scenarios, one is the fact that the body could be disrupted in the absorbing of vitamin D aka sun light or the person is just simply not getting enough sun light to replenish the lack of vitamin D within the body. In a sense we can look at the lack of vitamin D as a formation of photosynthesis within the body, just as a plant needs sunlight to help with the transformation of the water and carbon dioxide it needs as well as the nutrients it absorbs from the earth/dirt to change these substances to sugars so that the plant uses for a food source. Therefore we can look at the pancreas as needing the vitamin D in order to produce cells that will change the sugars consumed into a usable food source of muscles and the cells within the body to keep the organs healthy and functioning properly.

A list of food chemicals and how they can be linked to diseases such as diabetes:

- Sodium Benzoate: also known as benzoic acid European code is E211, this chemical substance approved by the FDA for antifungal effects as a food preservative is known to cause mitochondrial damage which can cause cell death and lead to cancer of serious neurological affects that can lead to DNA corruption causing a trigger for diabetes, its MSDS (Material safety data sheet) can be found here http://www.sciencelab.com/msds.php?msdsId=9927413

- Tartrazine aka common food dyes: The artificial food dye created from coal tar comes in all forms of colors such as red #3, and #40(E124), blue #1 and #2

(E133), Yellow #5 (E102) and #6 (E110) along with green which is based on curcumin extracted via petroleum products and propylene glycol, and White colorant which is created through titanium dioxide have been known to cause intestinal problems as well as severe asthma as well as cancer. Its MSDS sheet can be found here http://www.sciencelab.com/msds.php?msdsId=9927619

- BPA: BPA is bisphenol A is created through a petroleum based product and is used during the creation of most plastic bottles that cause a toxic effect after being left out in the sun which can cause death, It is actually cheaper to forgo adding BPA during the creation of plastic its MSDS can be found here http://www.cdhfinechemical.com/images/product/msds/37_2113175157_BisphenolA

[-CASNO-80-05-7-MSDS.pdf](#)

- BHT: (E320) also known as Butylated hydroxytoluene it can be found in pet foods, potato chips, nuts, noodles among other foods and is disguised as an antioxidant that is known to cause cancer and after long consumption can cause major damage to the intestinal track as well as super aging to the body and organs, its MSDS can be found here http://www.sciencelab.com/msds.php?msdsId=9923084

- BHA: (E320) Butylated hydroxyanisole Same as above affects it can be found in pet foods, potato chips, nuts, noodles among other foods and vegetable oils and is disguised as an antioxidant that is known to cause cancer and after long consumption can cause major damage to the intestinal track as well as super aging to the body and organs, its MSDS can be found here http://www.sciencelab.com/msds.php?msdsId=9923083

- TBHQ: tert-Butylhydroquinone can also be found in pet foods and many snack foods, and vegetable oils. There is no need for it; it is only used to protect foods from natural iron discoloration. It is usually found to be with BHA and BHT within foods and has been known to cause liver enlargement, neurotoxic effects, convulsions, and paralysis as well as vision disturbances, its MSDS can be found here http://www.sciencelab.com/msds.php?msdsId=9925167

- Polysorbates 80 and 20: a preservative found in many foods such as ice creams, it can be found in vaccinations and is highly dangerous, causing intestinal damage, sterility, and prevent nutrient absorbsion and can cause metabolic syndrome at the beginning of Diabetes type 2 The MSDS for Polysorbate

80 can be found here
http://www.sciencelab.com/msds.php?msdsId=9926645
and the MSDS for Polysorbate 20 can be found here
http://www.sciencelab.com/msds.php?msdsId=9926640

- Aspartame: An extremely dangerous sweetener that is actually 200 times sweeter than sugar and is found it all diet foods and drinks and will actually elevate the blood glucose levels in a person and can cause diabetic stress that can lead to hospitalization alternative names of this substance and where it can be found are Alternative names: Canderel, Tropicana Slim, NutraSweet, Equal, AminoSweet. Its MSDS can be found here http://www.sciencelab.com/msds.php?msdsId=9922975

- Splenda (AKA Sucralose): can cause blood glucose increases, gastrointestinal problems blurred vision and severe allergic reactions within a person, Splenda is not safe for cooking at all, once heated it undergoes a chemical change which makes its toxicity as dangerous as Agent Orange a chemical herbicide created for the Vietnam war and which is basically the same formula as today's round-up spray. The MSDS for Sucralose aka Splenda can be found here http://www.trade-chem.com/products/MSDS/sucralose.pdf

- Sucrose (AKA GMO beet sugars): Sucrose a genetically modified beet sugar which GMO or genetically modified means that it has been spliced down to the DNA level to include toxic pesticides and toxic herbicide resistance as well as bacteria that is used to help bond the substance together. Eating any genetically modified product can cause a genetic mutation within a person to trigger corrupted DNA and RNA to send negative information to the cells which can cause the development of autoimmune diseases that can lead to the development of diabetes and cancer. The MSDS can be found here http://www.sciencelab.com/msds.php?msdsId=9927285

- High Fructose Corn Syrup: HFCS a genetically modified corn syrup that causes metabolic syndrome to cause obesity in people, slowing down intestinal production, ingestion can lead to the development of cancer and as well diabetes type 1, its MSDS can be found here http://www.salvex.com/media/document/MSDS19.pdf

- Potassium Sorbate: is known to cause allergic reactions such as abdominal pain, sore throat, runny nose, itchy eyes it can be found in ice cream, cheese, yogurt, cereals and other snacks it has been linked to cancer, migraine headaches are a common symptom of potassium, sorbate poisoning from consumption, its msds can be found here http://www.agrovin.com/agrv/pdf/fichas_seguridad/antioxidantes/en/FDS_POTASSIUM_SORBATE_en.pdf

- Acesulfame K/Potassium: contains methylene chloride and is often found in protein powders, drinks, Jell-O, and many other diet foods and sodas, is often mixed with Splenda and aspartame to take away the bitter taste. It can cause respiratory diseases such as Asthma dizzy spells, memory loss abdominal cramping, aching joints, and dry skin eruptions. Its msds can be found here http://www.sciencelab.com/msds.php?msdsId=9922767

- Sodium/Potassium Fluoride: Fluoride the great lie that has been fed to the people for the development of easy mental control, causes abdominal problems skeletal fluorosis, dental fluorosis which is a pitting of the bones and teeth and stripping away of the enamel, but it also causes glucose intolerance which leads to type 1 diabetes and the destruction of the pancreas, Fluoride is extremely dangerous and causes many problems within the body, including mitochondrial DNA death. The msds for fluoride can be found here http://www.sciencelab.com/msds.php?msdsId=9927595

- Monosodium Glutamate: A food additive that is used for a flavor enhancer that is a neuro toxin that destroys the area of the brain that is linked to obesity which can lead to diabetes the msds for it can be found here https://static1.squarespace.com/static/54f0b505e4b017cb0d7a6f26/t/5568826ae4b01c525343b39a/1432912490560/USP+Monosodium+Glutamate+SDS.pdf
- Potassium Bromate: a category 2B carcinogen

meaning it causes cancer and has been banned in many areas throughout the world induces renal cell tumors, mesotheliomas of the peritoneum, and follicular cell tumors of the thyroid, this is mainly used in the bread making process. Its msds can be found here http://www.sciencelab.com/msds.php?msdsId=9927399

- Azodicarbonamide: A common bread additive this substance is also used for making flip flops and yoga

mats, can cause intestinal problems that can lead to gluten intolerance, blockage within the intestines can also lead to intestinal cancer. It can also cause respiratory problems and disrupt the immune system. When heated it creates a toxic by-product that can lead to major problems within the body. Its msds can be found here
http://www.sciencelab.com/msds.php?msdsId=9922989

- polyethylene glycol 400 and 3350: the scientific name for antifreeze, even though there is a food grade version of this substance it can cause major problems which can be linked to intestinal problems (abdominal cramps) it is known to cause liver damage and been linked to breast cancer, leukemia, brain and nervous system cancer, bladder cancer, stomach cancer and pancreatic cancer, as well as Hodgkin's disease. The msds for each one can be found here for the 400 http://www.sciencelab.com/msds.php?msdsId=9926620 and here for the 3350 http://www.sciencelab.com/msds.php?msdsId=9926625 Now that some of the substances have been identified that can cause autoimmune disease as well as break down of the liver and other organ functions we can move on to treatment for a possible cure for the causes of diabetes which will lead to a cure for diabetes itself. NOTE: if you are not prepared to change your diet completely none of this will work for you, and the excuse that organic foods are too expensive, ask yourself if you can continue paying the hospital bills, thus you see that the organic food and detox process is less expensive.

The first steps in the process of healing is knowing what one is dealing with, the second step is treating the problem and removal of everything that could possibly cause a problem within the body and the mind, both of which are important to the process of healing and detoxification.

What is detoxification: this is a process in which the toxins such as heavy metals and chemicals that are found in food preservatives as well as pesticides and herbicides are removed from the body to return the body to normal function. This process can be done through consumption of herbs, distilled water and colloidal silver; exercise must also be included in this process to help circulate the blood and help to wash the toxins out of the body.

Detox plan for curing the problems that cause diabetes, remember always ask about allergic reactions to herbs before giving any detox drink.

- Exercise at least 2 times a day 15 to 30 minutes at a time using a cardio workout in order to raise the heart rate and circulate the blood, first time either in the morning or afternoon then once before bed.

- Make sure you get plenty of sunlight, the natural increase of Vitamin D from the sun is important in recovering the health and improving the immune system

- The Use of Distilled water should be consumed within a 2 month period of time as well the distilled water should be used in all forms of herbal tea making to provide maximum benefits.

- Colloidal silver strength of ppm should be at least 30 to 150ppm in order to help cleans the toxins from the brain and heal the intestinal track and repair the nervous system. This is a bit lengthy of an explanation based on the way silver interacts with the body as a conductor to help in repair of the nervous system, removing the contaminated bacteria and destroying viruses within the body. It has been known to react to over 650 different pathogens causing substances such as aluminum to be removed from nervous system attachment and removing neural synapse disruption. This should be consumed 3 times a day dosage should be 1 shot glass full once in the morning, afternoon and once in the evening.

- The use of iodine supplements with the removal of fluoride and other toxic heavy metals and repair of the metabolic rate aka thyroid function,

- Avoid Microwave use completely.
- Herbal treatments for curing pancreas dysfunction as found through research treating pancreatic problems can be done through an herbal tea mixture of milk thistle, holy basil, ginger, dandelion and turmeric. Fennel Greek is also used as an herbal tea to help reduce levels of blood sugars.

(Jockers, D., Dr. (2018). 7

Strategies to Heal Pancreatitis Naturally) has an article listed about details on how to heal the pancreas naturally.

- Along with the herbal treatments for curing the pancreas one should consider the use of ORMUS/ORMES (Orbitally Rearranged Mono Atomic Elements) also known as white powder of gold, this will boost the healing of the body and repair of organs such as the pancreas

- Foods that can help lower the levels of sugar in the body for also beneficial for people that have high blood pressure due to elevated blood sugar levels such as Kale, Red Onion, carrot greens, beets can help with the elasticity of the blood veins if there are cardiac problems which helps to reduce blood pressure, Jamaica tea without sugar can help to lower the blood pressure by reducing the level of sugar in the blood, eggplant, nopales, verdolagas also known as wood sorrel which is in the family of clover, other herbs also cilantro, oregano, organic garlic powder, and organic onion powder can assist in a detox as well as cayenne pepper though very little bit is recommended due to its heat content. Bread products and pasta should be gluten free to eliminate high carbohydrates within the body for this Quinoa and amaranth is also recommended for a diet as well as Asparagus can help to regulate the blood sugar levels.

A proper diet plan for helping to heal diabetes and problems that cause diabetes should be followed using the foods and herbs listed here and everything must be consumed organically with absolutely no conventional or genetically modified foods or food chemicals. The elevation of sugar within the blood causes a raise in blood pressure if insulin is not created from the pancreas then the blood sugar levels can become toxic and it is necessary to use the detox diet. Every person must be consulted personally before providing them a diet to ensure that there are no adverse side-effects from the consumption of any of the foods listed, this is needed to prevent allergic reactions. A better controlled list of what can be consumed for a diet plan as well as what should be avoided will be placed down below:

Foods and herbs that can be used for healing diabetic problems:

1. Herbal teas for healing the pancreas milk thistle, holy

basil, ginger, dandelion and turmeric. A Fennel Greek tea can also be used to help lower blood sugar levels
2. Kale
3. Zucchini
4. Asparagus
5. Eggplant
6. Verdolagas also known as wood sorrel which is in the family of clover
7. Jamaica tea without sugar
8. Cilantro
9. Nopales
10. Garlic or garlic powder

11. Red Onion or onion powder
12. Quinoa
13. Amaranth
14. Gluten free pastas and breads (non-rice) must be made of corn and amaranth
15. Flaxseed
16. Brown rice can be consumed but in small quantities otherwise avoid completely
17. Cinnamon

Foods to avoid with diabetes

- Most fruits because of the natural high sugar content though sour cherries are okay
- Any high carbohydrate foods or artificial sweeteners though stevia, organic stevia is okay to use as a substitute if one needs sugar
- Absolutely anything processed, vegetables are best prepared fresh

- Honey, agave and any kind of sweetened drink other than the use of stevia
- Yogurt and any milk products
- Any high fat meats, so eating chicken or fish is best or lean meats, avoid pork completely as it causes intestinal damage and may be a cause of diabetic viral infection relations

This document has been completely researched in ways for helping to heal diabetes through possibly treating the main causes of diabetic problems, as well as possible solutions for healing the pancreas which is where the diabetic problems begin at due to an autoimmune disease or other problems listed here within this document.

Copyright @JLVreeland 2018 all rights reserved by Black Dragon KI Corporation

Personal progress notes

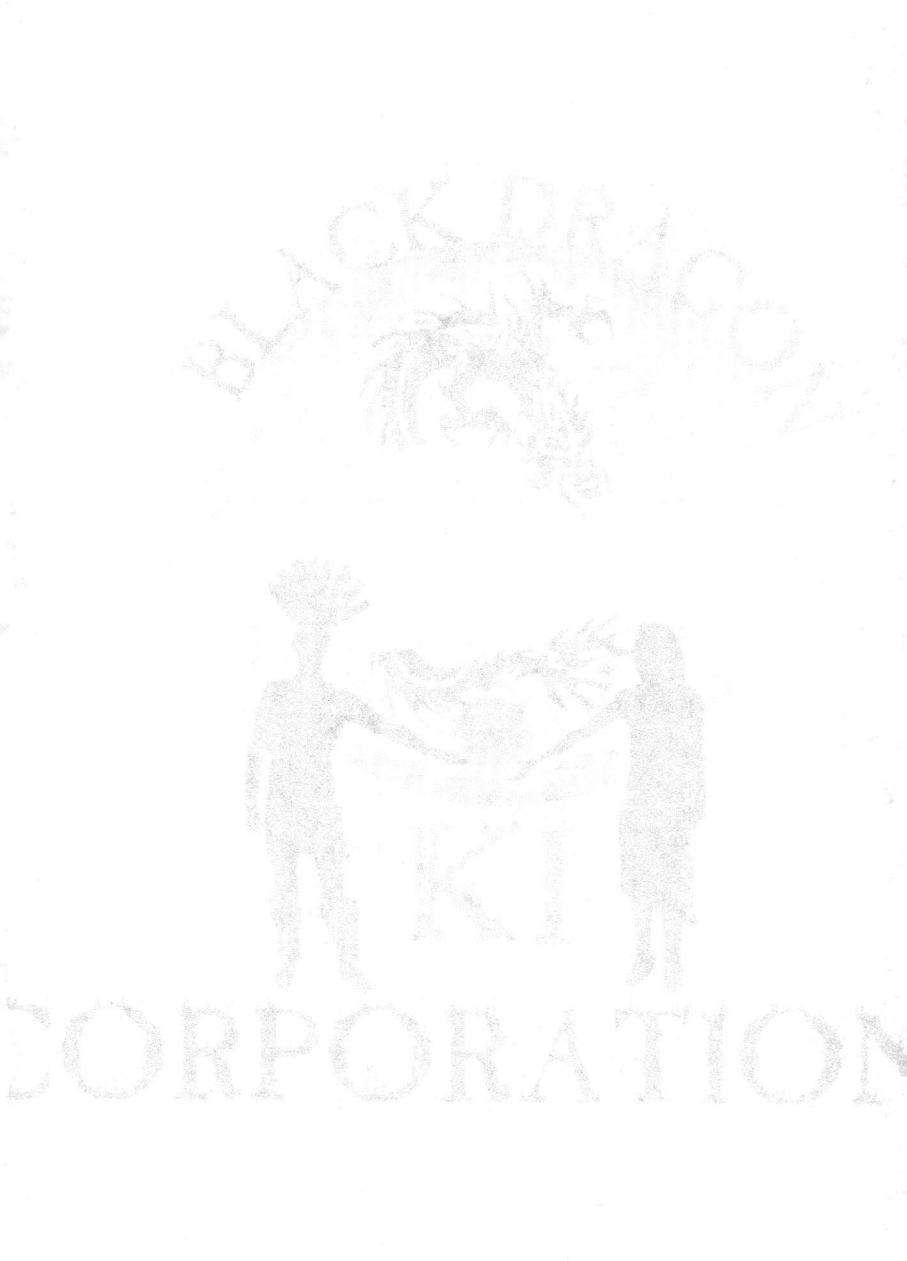

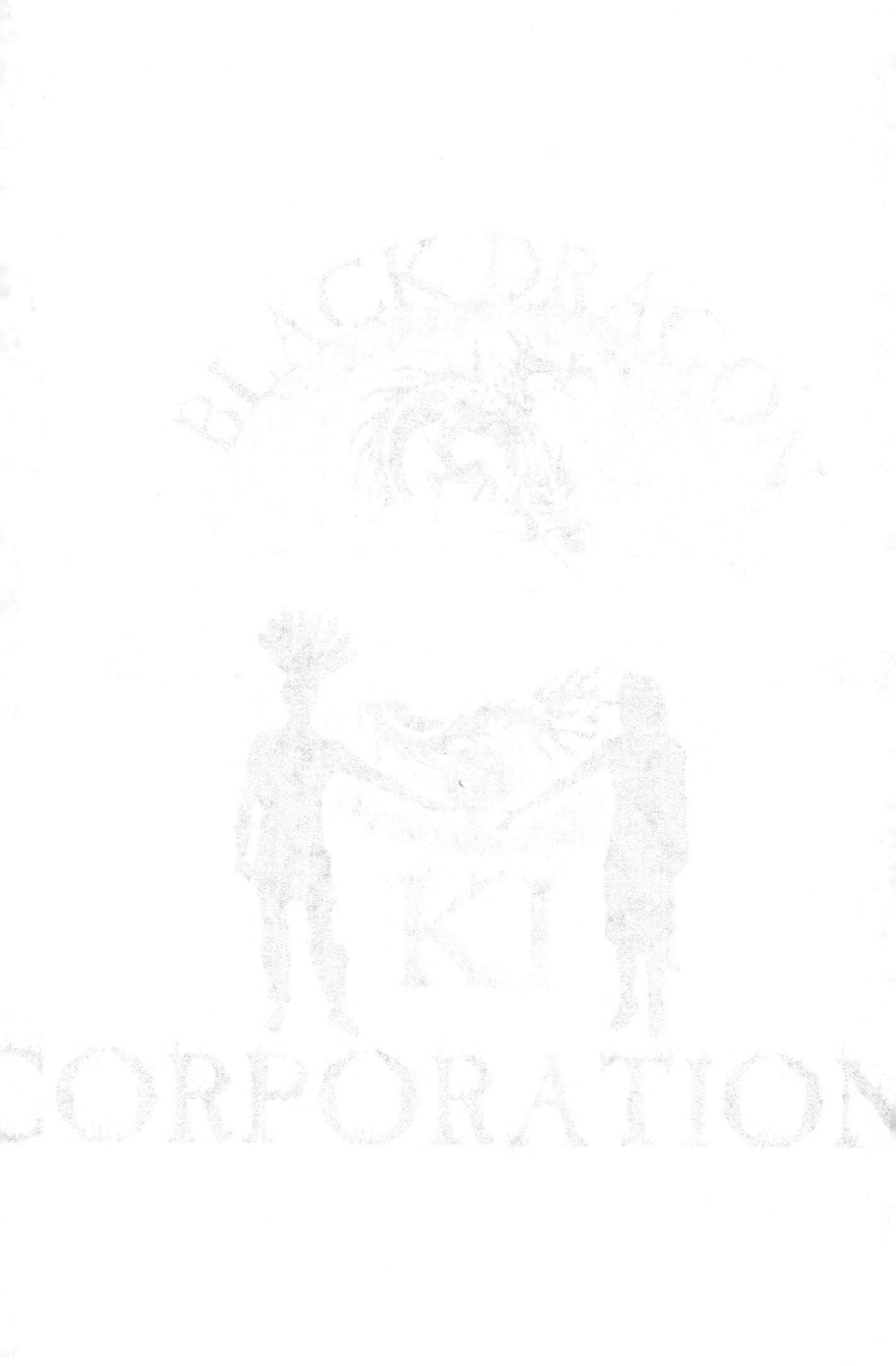

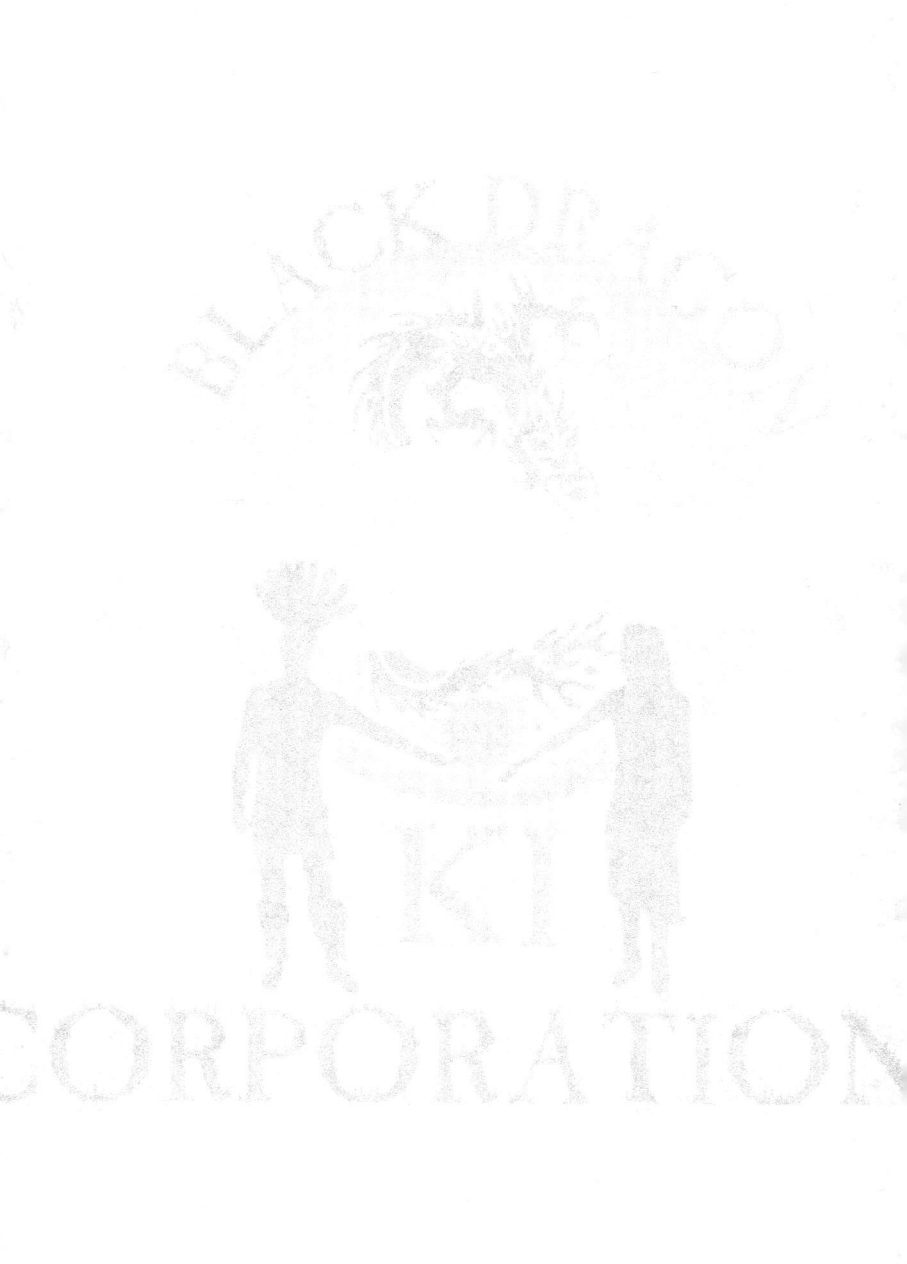

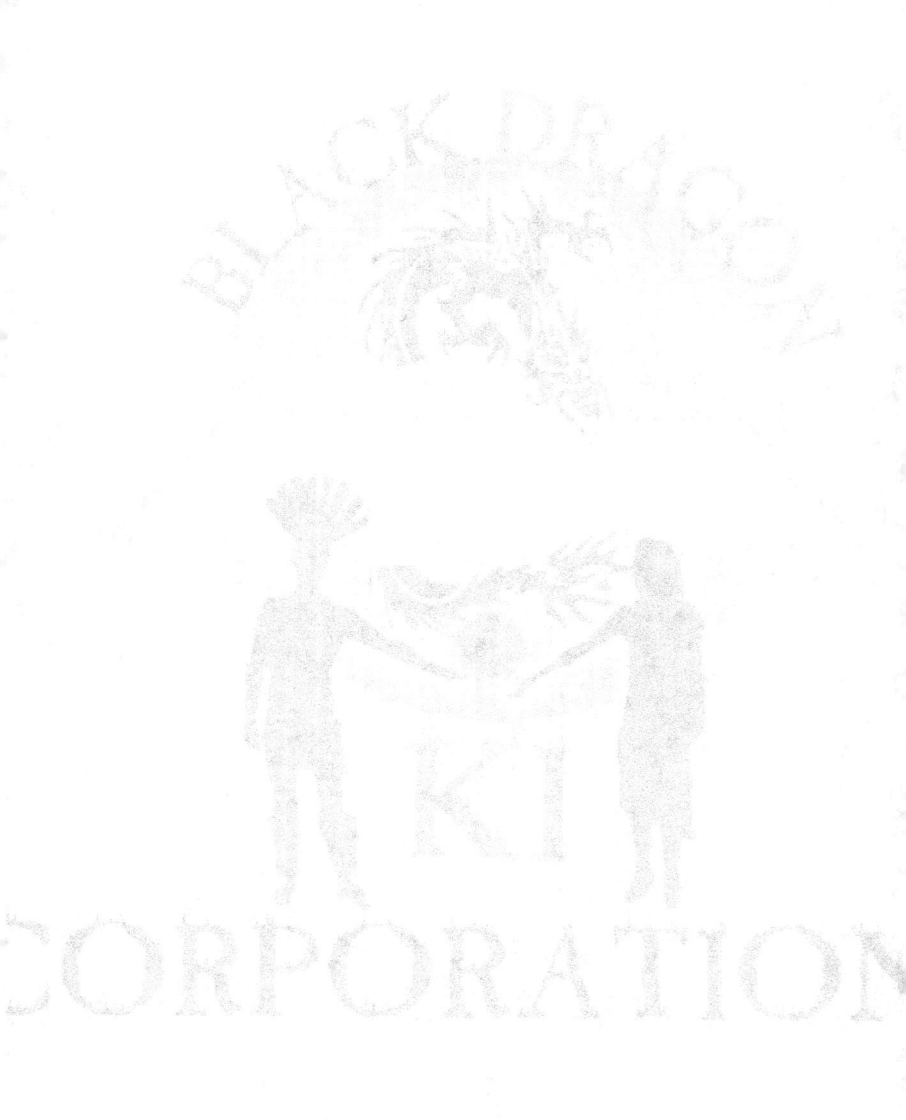

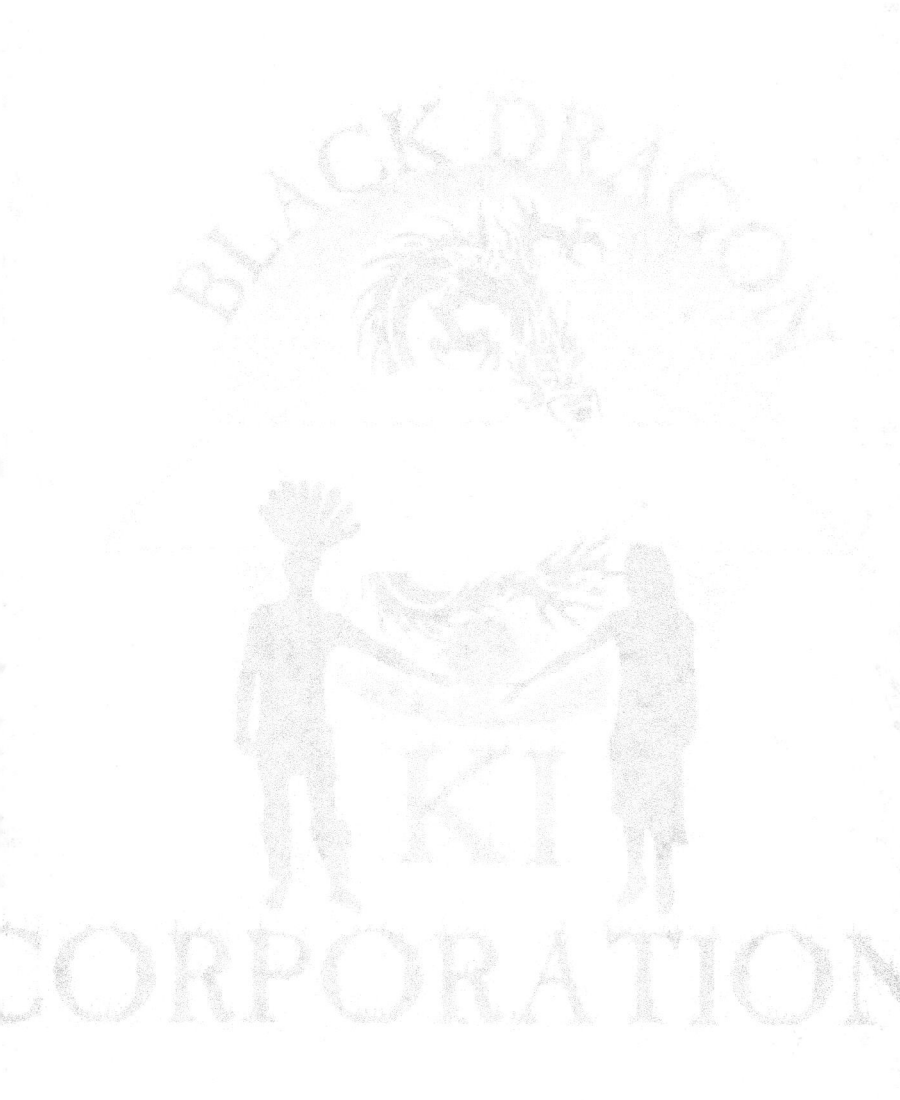

References for type 1 diabetes:

Type 1 diabetes (2016, May 09) Retrieved February 25, 2018, from https://www.nhs.uk/conditions/type-1-diabetes/

Wolters Kluwer Health, Inc. (2007, February 01).This is the 360 Link Sidebar Helper frame - use this to find other links to this content or links to additional library resources. Retrieved February 25, 2018

References for type 2 diabetes:

NHS (2016, June 27). Type 2 diabetes Retrieved February 25, 2018, from https://www.nhs.uk/conditions/type-2-diabetes/#causes-of-type-2-diabetes

American Diabetes Association (1995) Type 2 Retrieved February 25, 2018, from http://www.diabetes.org/diabetes-basics/type-2/?referrer=https%3A%2F%2Fwww.google.com.mx%2F

McCulloch, D. K. MD Diabetes mellitus Retrieved February 25, 2018, from https://www.uptodate.com/contents/diabetes-mellitus-type-2-overview-beyond-the-basics

Herbs for healing the pancreas as well as learning about pancreas functions

Jockers, D., Dr. (2018) 7 Strategies to Heal Pancreatitis Naturally Retrieved

February 26, 2018, from

https://drjockers.com/pancreatitis/

www.ingramcontent.com/pod-product-compliance
Lightning Source LLC
Chambersburg PA
CBHW052339220526
45472CB00001B/497